Vegan Keto

by Madison Green

Table of Contents

What is Keto?

Keto is short for ketosis, a metabolic state where your body burns ketones for energy, as opposed to the natural state of glycolysis where your body burns glucose for energy. Your next question is probably, what does that even mean? To understand what ketosis is, and why keto is such a popular and effective diet, we must start with a little biology lesson.

Your body consumes food for energy. Yes, it's true. I know, I was also shocked when I first found out. Your stomach acid and stomach enzymes breakdown the carbohydrates and starches you consume into glucose which is absorbed by your stomach and intestines into your blood stream, fueling every cell in your body[1]. Excess glucose is turned into lipids which are stored in fat cells as fat.

On a keto diet, you induce ketosis in your body. The keto diet is punctuated by a rigid structure of high-fat and low-carb foods. When your body recognizes it is not receiving enough glucose to survive, it enters ketosis. During ketosis, your liver turns fat into ketones through a process called ketogenesis and replaces the glucose with said ketones in your blood stream[2]. Effectively, your body chemistry completely changes and directly uses stored fat for energy instead of glucose.

Unless you've been living under a small boulder for the past several years, there is a very good chance you've heard of the keto diet and that's why you bought this book. It seems like everyone is talking about this new diet craze, even though it was invented in the 1920's to treat pediatric epilepsy[3]. A-List celebrities from Katie Couric and Gwyneth Paltrow to Lebron James and Tim Tebow have all gushed about the benefits of the keto diet. But if it was invented in the 1920's, why are we only hearing about it now?

The ketogenic diet effectively vanished from medicine shortly after its invention because of the advent of effective anticonvulsant drugs[4]. Remember, the keto diet was not originally intended for weight loss but to treat epilepsy in children. With effective medication, there wasn't a need for patients to dramatically change their diets. For 70 years, there wasn't a peep or a study about the revolutionary diet. In the 1990's, Hollywood producer Jim Abrahams (*Airplane!*, *The Naked Gun*, and *Kentucky Fried Movie*) brought the diet back into the public consciousness after it helped his son with his epilepsy. Abrahams started the Charlie Foundation to raise awareness for the keto diet[5]. Still, this doesn't explain why the keto diet became so popular only a couple years ago and not in the 1990's.

Did celebrities like the Kardashians popularize the diet, or did the popularity of the diet draw their attention? The most likely cause for the explosive popularity of the keto diet seems to be Instragram. On the 'Gram as it were, you can find countless, mind blowing body transformations of people who used the keto diet to lose weight. When you combine the age of Facebook and Instagram with a diet that actually works, popularity was inevitable. Combine that with celebrities who have found success with the diet without even being paid to endorse it; now you have a bonafide phenomenon.

Why Keto Works

At this point you might be thinking, whatever happened to those other fad diets, like Atkin's and Paleo? Isn't this just another fad? That's a very good, and very important question. To the uneducated, keto diet looks exactly like the Atkin's diet. While they are both low-carb diets, Atkin's tends to focus on protein, while Keto focuses on fat, and for a very good reason. Keto actually works with a wealth of studies to back it up. It is indisputable that not only does ketosis exist, but it can be induced through diet, and it makes your body burn fat for energy. This hard science alone places keto above every other diet ever created.

Every year, biologists learn more about how our body metabolizes food. And what they've found out recently is the mechanisms in the keto diet are conducive to massive weight loss. Everyone use to "know" weight loss was as simple as burning more calories than you intake. Now we know the body could never be so simple.

As it turns out, insulin has a massive affect on the ability of our body to use glucose and burn fat. Insulin does many things in our body, mainly signaling to our cells to absorb the glucose in our bloodstream. Insulin also sends chemical signals to our fat cells to pick up the lipids in our blood stream and to retain the fat we already have[6]. But with the keto diet, we never consume enough carbs to the point our insulin levels become a problem. Our body uses ketones for energy instead, and our fat cells release fat to be burned.

Another thing biologists have discovered is a neuro-transmitter called orexin. Orexin creates a feeling of wakefulness in our brain. It should come as no shock that people on the keto diet boast about their new found energy levels. Not only are their bodies burning massive amounts of energy, but there is plenty of orexin produced in their brain. It's very common for us to turn to a soda or sugary coffee for energy in the afternoon, but biologists have discovered that protein triggers the production of orexin, not sugar[7]. And this emphasis on protein also plays into the keto diet.

The Keto Diet

Now that I have thoroughly piqued your interest in the keto diet, the most important part is, what exactly is the diet? The keto diet is a high-fat, low-carb diet similar to Atkins, but much more effective. The great secret to the keto diet is the 5% rule. The only way for the keto diet to work is to reduce the amount of carbs you consume to just 5% of your total calorie intake. This rule is unbreakable if you want to lose weight. If you can't reduce your calories from carbohydrates to 5% of your total diet, your body will not enter ketosis, and you will not lose weight. Remember, this diet is not predicated on calorie counting. Calories do not matter on the keto diet. The only thing that matters is inducing ketosis, and the only way to do that is to reduce the carbs in your diet to 5% or less.

You can do your own research, but the generally accepted rule for the keto diet is that your diet should be 75% fat, 20% protein, and 5% carbs by calorie[8].

Remember, you're not counting calories here, just your ratio of calories. And it cannot be stressed enough how important that 5% rule is. Without 5% carbs, you will not lose weight, plain and simple. The
entire point of the keto diet is to restrict the number of carbs you consume to the point your entire body chemistry changes. It simply will not change if it gets enough carbs to function on glucose. This isn't about starving yourself. You're literally allowed to pig out on fatty foods to your heart's content while on the keto diet.

What's With All These Diets?

If you scoped out the table of contents, you may have noticed that we're going to cover not just the vegan keto diet, but also the vegetarian keto diet, and the basic keto diet. Make no mistake, this is a book about the vegan keto diet, but the vegan keto diet is a very difficult diet to adhere to. In the vegan keto diet section, we'll discuss the diet at length but also go over how it's a diet for your mind as well. Diet's are never just about food portions and selections. No diet can succeed if you don't have the willpower to adhere to it. That has never been truer than on keto. Because the goal of keto is to induce ketosis, and the only way to induce ketosis is by restricting your carb intake to just 5%, there is no room for error. The diet simply does not work without ketosis. One of the great things about keto that separates it from all other diets aside from the hard, provable science is that you get to eat whatever you want as long as you obey the 5% rule. But that means if you don't obey the 5% rule, you won't lose any weight at all. There are no cheat days. Your willpower will play a bigger factor in the keto diet than in any other diet

Now you compound the restrictiveness of the keto diet with the restrictions of a vegan diet, and you have one of the most challenging diets known to man. I don't want you going into this diet thinking things will be easy. Remember, your willpower will be tested like it has never been tested before. You have to eat every single day, multiple times a day. That means every day, multiple times a day your willpower will be tested. The vegan keto diet offers the greatest of difficulties but also the greatest of rewards: a healthy, ethical diet guaranteed to help you lose weight if it is adhered to. It all comes down to your willpower. I am giving you all the knowledge required to complete a vegan keto diet, but where my knowledge ends, your willpower begins. Knowledge can temper your willpower. Nothing shakes your will to succeed like sudden, immensely difficult challenges. I don't want that to happen to you. I want you to go into this with the most realistic expectations, so you can mentally prepare for the challenges you face. Realistic expectations are one of the most important ways to temper your willpower.

I can almost guarantee you will fail...at first. No one is a perfect dieter. No one ever achieved perfection on their first attempt. You ever see the first season of *The Simpsons*? Perfection does not come immediately. As someone who has lost substantial weight in her life, I can tell you the greatest secret to weight loss is, **never give up**. I know that seems a little obvious or pedantic, but hear me out. Many dieters enter a diet with the best of intentions. Inevitably, they will make a mistake or have a moment of weakness.

It can be as simple as grabbing a former go-to snack without realizing it's not vegan-keto, or maybe your body is craving something sugary or fatty and you indulge
. You could have a rough day at work or face a break up, and all you want to do is turn to a pint of ice cream for solace. That's okay. You're not a failure for showing weakness. We all have our moments of weakness. That's what makes us human. The most important thing you can do, the secret to dieting success, is to restart and try again.

If you grab those potato chips or candy bar in a moment of weakness, if you crack open a beer after work without thinking, the most important thing you can do is try harder the next day. And if you mess up again, try harder the next day. You will get better. Some of us will have a moment of weakness, or a bad day, or even a bad week, but if you try again the next time, if you commit yourself to making it work, you will eventually succeed. Ask any fighter, and they will tell you they learn more from their losses than from their wins. Your losses will teach you the foods and situations to avoid. If you resort to alcohol to relax, maybe next time volunteer to be the designated driver when you go out with friends. If you come home from work and eat junk food because you don't know what you want to eat, write up meal plans you can stick to. **Every failure is an opportunity to be better.** Not only do you learn from your mistakes, but you temper your willpower. You teach your mind and body that not only can you overcome your mistakes, but you can come out even stronger. It may seem silly, but dieting will teach you exactly the kind of person you are. And I bet you'll find out you have more strength and willpower than you ever thought possible.

For some of us, vegan keto is not a viable diet choice. But the only way to find out is to try it. In *Vegan Keto*, I give you all the information and meal plans you need to succeed. But even then, sometimes that's not enough. We each have our own levels of willpower. Sometimes our lives are too stressful, or our doctor advises us against a vegan keto diet, or we don't have the money, or maybe we don't have the market to purchase the vegan keto food we need. That's nothing to be ashamed of. **You are not an inferior person because you failed at your diet**. Not every diet is right for every person. If there was such a diet, then everyone would already be on it. As the great Jean-Luc Picard so eloquently put it, "*It is possible to commit no mistakes and still lose. That is not a weakness. That is life.*"

In this book, I'm giving you several dietary guidelines you can follow based on your current situation. *Vegan Keto* is obvious dedicated to a vegan ketogenic diet, but as stated, it's one of the most difficult diets to adhere to. I don't want you to feel like a failure because you couldn't adhere to such a difficult diet. That's why I'm including information on veganism, vegetarianism, vegetarian keto, and the standard keto diet. While I cannot make any guarantees about weight loss for vegans and vegetarians, I can say that if you follow a vegetarian keto or standard keto diet correctly, you will lose weight. I don't want you failing a vegan keto diet then regretting you bought this book. My two main goals are to give you the knowledge and motivation you need to be healthier, and making sure you are absolutely glad you bought this book.

I can tell you right now that vegetarian keto is much MUCH easier than vegan keto when you're allowed to add eggs, cheese, butter, and cream to your food.

These high fat foods are ideal for the keto diet, and many would argue are immensely satisfying. If you're a vegan, I know it can sound disgusting to eat animal fat and ovum from animals who probably live in horrible conditions, but remember that grass fed dairy products exist, as well as pasture eggs where the chickens can roam free. We will discuss the ethics of veganism in the vegan vs. vegetarian section later, but many people gravitate towards veganism out of respect for animals. There is definitely a balance between ethical food consumption and effective weight loss, and much of it will be determined by your personal principles, willpower, financial situation, market availability, and medical history.

Even easier than a vegetarian keto diet is the basic keto diet. If you're a vegan you'll probably want to skip this section about meat and animal products. For those who have found that veganism and vegetarianism does not work for them, you can still absolutely lose weight on a standard keto diet. Combining eggs, cheese, butter, and cream with fatty meats like pork belly, pork shoulder, ribs, ribeye, bacon, chicken thighs, and chicken wings make for one exciting diet. Yes, you get to eat all that delicious fatty food on keto. Remember, keto is never about cutting calories. You are simply reducing your caloric intake from carbs to 5% of your diet. After that, you get to eat whatever you want. This is a huge reason why keto is so popular. Just be following the 5% rule, you literally get to feast like a king every night.

Vegan keto is not designed to test your willpower. This is not some impossible task set before you. The goal is to lose weight. If you cannot adhere to a vegan keto diet or a vegetarian keto diet, there is no shame in the standard keto diet. As long as you are losing weight in a sane manner under a doctor's supervision, there is no wrong way to lose the weight. And who doesn't want to eat bacon while they lose weight?

Please never, EVER condescend to someone about their diet choices. You do not know what an individual is going through when you see them eating a bacon cheeseburger or when they ask for vegan menu options. The same way you probably hate people stereotyping vegans, the same is true for meat eaters who hate when vegans condescend to them. People get mad at each other for the most insane things anymore. Wearing yoga pants to school, serving coffee in a red cup, casting women in a movie, putting dijon mustard on a burger, eating pizza with a knife and fork. I think it's about time we all calm down. If you see someone eating a fat BLT or making a 12 egg omelette, don't get mad. They might not have the knowledge of factory farm life that you have. They may not be as sympathetic to animals as you. They might not have the financial resources to buy vegan food, which is not cheap compared to meat and junk food. They might not have access to a store that even sells vegan food. Their life choices are not your responsibility. And it is not your responsibility to go up and educate them. If you want to educate people on veganism, start a blog, write a book, start your own Youtube channel. That way the people who are interested in veganism can learn more about it. You're not going to win people over by shaming them or yelling at them. You must agree to disagree.

And the same thing goes with you carnivores. Vegans have made a very difficult choice to abstain from animal products. Eating a salad or drinking soy milk is not a great reason to mock someone.

The amount of noise their car engine makes is not indicative of their sexuality. These diets are not an excuse to condescend to someone who does not eat like you or does not have the willpower you have. I think a pretty safe statement is we would all like to at least be a little healthier. Keto is an amazing way for almost any person to become healthier. Whether you are a vegan, vegetarian, or enjoy gnawing the bones of animals, we can all get to a healthier place. We don't know how much money someone has, what their life is like, how much information they received, or what they aspire to. Let's not judge each other for our diet choices. I absolutely want you to share this book with friends and family members. I want you to blog and vlog about how it has helped you and others. But don't push it on a stranger because you see them enjoying a rack of ribs or a milkshake. They will only get to the level of health they desire when they choose to take the first step. Harassing them won't get them there.

The Numerous Health Benefits of Keto

The keto diet can help you do more than just lose weight, though it is very powerful in that regard. Because of the nature of a restrictively low-carb diet like keto, you can expect several, incidental health improvements to go along with it.

Firstly, you will reduce your risk of heart disease. High levels of blood sugar cause damage to our blood vessels. And that same blood sugar can also damage the nerves that regulate our heart beat. It is well established chronically high blood sugar is a danger to our heart health[9]. But with the keto diet, we never have to worry about the correlation between blood sugar and heart health because we've effectively eliminated our blood sugar levels and replaced it with ketone levels. Even if you don't need to lose weight, the keto diet is an excellent way to protect your heart.

Secondly, the keto diet has been proven as an effective cancer treatment. Yes, it's true. Multiple studies have proven that the keto diet is an extremely effective diet for those battling cancer. Because of the unique nature of the diet, there are several mechanisms in your body that occur under ketosis that incidentally fight cancer. First off, cancer feeds off the glucose in your body. Without glucose, the cancer grows much slower than usual. But under ketosis, you don't have any glucose in your blood stream, and this starves the cancer. Incidentally, because you don't have blood sugar, your insulin levels are very low, another body chemistry that screws up cancer's ability to spread. Finally, a keto diet eliminates the visceral fat stored in your gut. There is a strong correlation between levels of visceral fat and rates of cancer. Keto eliminates this fat[10].

Thirdly, keto is an extremely effective treatment for many neurological disorders. From Alzheimer's, to Parkinson's, and epilepsy, keto is one of the most effective forms of treatment[11]. We have known for almost a century that keto can treat epilepsy in children, but what scientists are finding out now is that many symptoms of neurological disorders can be curbed as well. Keto massively ramps up the amount of calories you burn, and that's doubly true for your brain. The working theory is that ketones provide a massive amount of energy for the brain as well as stabilized the neurons damaged by these diseases[11].

And to top it all off, researchers have found that the keto diet may be effective in reducing acne[12]. It's hard to believe that one simple diet could have so many health benefits, but it really just goes to prove how powerful the diet is. When a diet is based in hard science and has real, measurable effects on your body, it is inevitable it would come with multiple health benefits. Keto isn't about starving yourself. You can literally eat whatever you want. All keto is, is a simple 5% rule that will completely change your life. But I bet you want more than that. I bet you want to know how to combine such a powerful diet with a sane and moral food consumption philosophy. Well, aren't you lucky you found this book. In ***Vegan Keto***, you will learn everything you wanted to know about the keto diet and how to combine it with a vegan lifestyle. Not only will you learn the rules and ways of the diet, but the underlying philosophy of a vegan lifestyle and why so many people are drawn to it. Included in the book is a two week diet plan complete with a plethora of snack and dessert options. That's right, you get to eat dessert every night on the vegan keto diet. It would be unethical not to include a list of side effects that come with a keto diet. No diet is 100% safe for everyone, and you should always consult a doctor before making any dramatic changes to your diet. We will discuss the dangerous ketoacidosis and why you really don't need to worry about it at all since it is incredibly rare.

This is your first step to a brave new world where you control your weight and health with a powerful diet grounded in hard science. Are you ready to take the first step? The book is in your hands, all you have to do is turn the page and begin.

1. Kaiser Permanente, *How Our Bodies Turn Food Into Energy*, McCulloch, David, MD, March 2014, https://wa.kaiserpermanente.   org/healthAndWellness?item=%2Fcommon%2FhealthAndWellness%2Fconditions%2Fdiabetes%2FfoodProcess.html

2, 3, 4, 5. Wikipedia, *Ketogenic Diet*, https://en.wikipedia.org/wiki/Ketogenic_diet#Diet

6. Healthline, *4 Ways Sugar Can Make You Fat* Gunnars, Kris February 4, 2013 https://www.healthline.com/nutrition/4-ways-sugar-makes-you-fat

7. Science Daily *Mid-afternoon slump? Why a sugar rush may not be the answer* University of Cambridge November 29, 2011 https://www.sciencedaily.com/releases/2011/11/111116124714.htm

8. Healthline, *The Ketogenic Diet: A Detailed Beginner's Guide to Keto*, Mawer, Rudy, July 2018, https://www.healthline. com/nutrition/ketogenic-diet-101

9. National Institute of Diabetes and Digestive and Kidney Diseases, *Diabetes, Heart Disease, and Stroke* Buse, John B. M.D. Ph.D. https://www.niddk.nih.gov/health-information/diabetes/overview/preventing-problems/heart-disease-stroke

10. Healthline, *Can the Keto Diet Help Fight Cancer?* Fischer, Kristen October 2018 https://www.healthline.com/health-news/can-the-keto-diet-help-fight-cancer

11. Science Daily, *Ketogenic Diet Prevents Seizures By Enhancing Brain Energy Production, Increasing Neuron Stability* Emory University Health Sciences Center, November 2005, https://www.sciencedaily.com/releases/2005/11/051114220938.htm

12. The National Center for Biotechnology Information, *Nutrition and acne: therapeutic potential of ketogenic diets.* Paoli A, Grimaldi K, Toniolo L, Canato M, Bianco A, Fratter A. February 2012, https://www.ncbi.nlm.nih.gov/pubmed/22327146

Veganism vs. Vegetarianism: What's the difference?

Veganism

Veganism is a way of life where an individual abstains from using animal products as frequently as possible but within reason, especially as it pertains to food, clothing, and products tested on animals[1,2]. For our purposes we are going to focus exclusively on the diet and general philosophy of veganism, as many people choose veganism over vegetarianism for the ethical implications, not necessarily for the diet choices. Abstaining from the consumption of animal products means a vegan is not allowed consume any meat, including fish, frogs, roe, crustaceans (crab, lobster, crawfish), arthropods (shrimp, prawn), mollusks (clams, mussels, oysters, scallops, snails, squid, octopus, abalone), and sea cucumber (as it turns out, sea cucumber is an animal and not a cucumber, someone really screwed up). This prohibition on animal products goes beyond meat though. Vegans are not allowed to consume eggs, milk, cheese, yogurt, mayonnaise, honey, whey or kefir (a fermented milk drink, not to be confused with tibicos made in a similar way from grains and is actually vegan).

As you can see, no one gets into veganism for the delightful array of food options. The western diet is based on many food staples that would never be considered vegan. Veganism is strictly for health and ethical reasons. Many people find it difficult to stick to a vegan diet, but those who do say the physical and emotional payoff is well worth it. There are many staples of the vegan diet that are required to make up for the lack of nutrients in vegan food. It may seem strange that a plant based diet would ever lack in nutrients, but critical diet components like protein, calcium, and omega-3 fatty acids are absent from many vegan diets. That is why vegans rely on food staples to ensure they never lack for nutrition.

Soy Protein

Protein is such a critical part of your health that it cannot be overstated. From your skin, hair, and muscle health to general brain function and the strength of your immune system, every part of your body relies on protein. Your body literally needs protein to create new cells and survive[3]. Because vegans completely abstain from meat, adequate protein can be difficult to consume on a daily basis. But despite common misconception, vegans actually have a plethora of protein options.

The go-to protein for vegans has always been soy. Soy beans, also know as edamame, has 17 grams of protein in just one cup. That's more than a standard 1/8th pound burger patty. Not to be outdone, tofu and tempeh both have 16-19 grams of protein per serving. But miso laughs at such a pathetic display, coming in at a whopping 32 grams of protein in just 1 cup! That's more than a quarter pound beef patty.

Tofu is coagulated soy milk where the milk curds are pressed into cubes and can be used for virtually anything.

You can fry it in a pan, grill it, or even use it as an egg substitute in omelettes and quiches. My favorite is spicy tofu fried with mushrooms, but your options are virtually limitless. Tempeh is fermented soy beans, but shouldn't be confused with miso as the products look and taste completely different. Tempeh kind of looks like those to-go cereal bars as you can see the individual soy beans in the tempeh cake. While tofu has a very neutral flavor, tempeh has a mushroom-like, earthy flavor that can become powerful if aged. Miso is a fermented soybean paste most often used as a flavoring ingredient instead of the main piece of the meal. It is made by fermenting soybeans with salt and koji, a special type of fungus. Miso is extremely salty and sometimes has a slightly sour taste to it. Bear in mind these are not simply soybeans left to rot just because they are fermented. Like wine, cheese, and sauerkraut, tempeh and miso are fermented under controlled conditions so their flavor and food safety can be controlled.

Many nutritionists argue miso and tempeh are much safer for you than tofu. I cannot recommend any food or diet options to you without informing you of the risks involved. Again, whenever making a massive change to your diet, always consult a doctor. Tofu is high in a chemical called phyto-estrogen, which is basically estrogen derived from plants. Consuming too much phyto-estrogen can have serious negative effects on your health. In women, elevated estrogen levels have been linked to infertility, breast cancer, and a lowered sex drive. In men, elevated estrogen levels can cause gynecomastia (where the man grows breasts), mood swings, and erectile dysfunction. I want to be perfectly blunt that eating tofu will not give you cancer, but consuming large amounts of phyto-estrogen is not safe for your health.

Tempeh and miso on the other hand are not high in phyto-estrogen. This is because phytates are broken down during the fermentation process. Not only are these fermented products easier to digest, but you no longer run the risk of consuming too much phyto-estrogen[4]. And let us not forget that aside from quinoa, soy is the only vegan food that forms a complete protein.

Nuts, Legumes, and Seeds, Oh My!

Nuts are another staple of the vegan diet. From cashews and pecan, to peanuts, walnuts, and hazelnuts, to almonds and pistachios, nuts are highly nutritious as well as highly available. Nuts are a perfect vegan food because they combine a good source of protein, anywhere from 6-12 grams in a 1 oz. serving, with many essential vitamins and minerals such as iron, fiber, magnesium, and zinc[5]. In addition to adequate protein, vegans must also focus intensely on their iron intake. Meats are rich in iron, so it is rare for someone with a western diet to have an iron deficiency. The same cannot be said for vegans. While vegans are no more at risk for iron deficiency anemia than meat eaters, they generally have lower levels of iron in their blood which is a risk factor for anemia[6]. Consuming Iron rich foods like nuts, brocoli, and spinach, along with vitamin-C rich foods is the key to avoiding iron deficiency. A struggle with the vegan diet is that certain vegan foods cause your body to resist nutrient absorption. That is why consuming vitamin-C with your iron rich foods is so important.

Not only are nuts a staple food, but nut spreads and butters are also delicious vegan treats that can be used in a variety of dishes.

Peanut butter is vegan except on the rare occasion that they decide to add honey to it. Almond butter is also a vegan treat if you want to mix things up. It should be said that Nutella is not vegan as it contains whey and milk. But still, nut butter allows you to create many a tasty snack. One of my all-time favorite snacks is slicing an apply then dipping the slices in peanut butter. You can also slather celery in peanut butter then sprinkle raisins on it for the classic ants-on-a-log. This book comes with two weeks of vegan keto recipes, I just like to gush about my favorite snacks.

Legumes are also an excellent source of protein for those looking to go vegan. Before you assume I made a huge mental misstep, I know peanuts are technically legumes, and you think maybe they should be down here. But let me holler at you. Peanuts are consumed like nuts, and peanut butter is used as nut butter. Remember the classic adage, *intelligence is knowing that peanuts are legumes, wisdom is knowing not to put them in three-bean salad*. Beans, lentils, and peas are all recognized as *real* legumes, and possess anywhere from 10-20 grams of protein per cup when cooked. These little nubs are rich in iron and zinc, but also problematic antinutrients. Antinutrients are compounds that occur naturally in plants and inhibit your body's absorption of certain vitamins and minerals. Antinutrients are one of the main downsides to a plant-based diet. Studies have proven you absorb nutrients at a more efficient rate with meat in your diet than with no meat. As stated previously, I will give you all the facts when entering into this diet. It would be irresponsible of me to conceal the real problem antinutrients pose to people on plant-based diets. Fortunately for us though, antinutrients can be overcome with a proper diet. When consuming yummy legumes, always full cook them, ferment them, or sprout them in order to breakdown the antinutrients. Never consume calcium rich foods with your legumes as the calcium binds to the iron and zinc and makes it more difficult for your body to absorb them. To counteract the effects of antinutrients, consume legumes with vitamin-C to help you absorb the zinc and iron more efficiently[7].

Before I close the book on legumes, I would be remissed if I didn't inform you of the wonders of beans and rice. When these two magical foods are combined, they form a complete protein. You see, nutrition facts are a bit misleading. Yes all these plants are rich in proteins, but it's a little more complicated than that. Protein is made up of 20 different amino acids. As should be obvious, a plant protein is very different from a moo-cow protein. That's because all animal protein is made from the 20 different amino acids your body needs. Unfortunately, almost no plants contain all 20 essential amino acids. Only edamame and quinoa hold that glorious distinction. One of the key components of a vegan diet is to gather protein from many different sources so the amino acids overlap until they form a complete protein. And as if some vegan god made it so, the delicious combination of beans and rice formed a complete set of amino acids all along.

Now settle down. I know you're super excited to get to the seeds. Vegans rely on a battery of seeds to meet their nutritional needs from sunflower and pumpkin seeds, to chia, flax, and hemp seeds (not that kind of hemp, I thought you were cool, man). Seeds are rich in protein, but also rich in fatty acids crucial to a healthy and functioning nervous system. Hemp seeds are easily the most nutritious of the lot with 9 grams of protein per 1 oz. serving. They also have an ideal ratio of omega-3 to omega-6 fatty acids[8]. Chia and flax seeds are rich in alpha-linolenic acid which your body can convert into other fatty acids such as EPA and DHA. EPA and DHA are generally only found in fish, so it's super important that vegans find an alternative source to these fatty acids.

Vegan Protein Power from Protein Powder!

Even with the previously mentioned foods, vegans can struggle to consume an adequate amount of protein. Fortunately for them, vegan protein shakes exist. Vegan protein shakes are made from plants such as soy, rice, hemp, or peanuts instead of whey like in traditional protein shakes. These protein powders can be used as meal substitutes or to supplement your protein intake. Please bear in mind that as stated previously, only the soy based protein shake has the complete set of amino acids your body needs. If you are not consuming a soy shake, then you should combine the powder with other protein sources to complete the set of amino acids. These powders can be added to smoothies or oat meal along with nut butter to offset the missing amino acids. Some people complain about the aftertaste of vegan protein powder, but that can be remedied with baking spices such as cinnamon, ginger, or nutmeg. Even vanilla and cacao can help with the taste. I'm including a link to a list of the highest rated vegan protein shakes so you can decide which one fits your needs the best[9].

Calcium and Choline

Calcium and Choline are two essential nutrients that vegans often struggle to consume enough of. While cheese, milk, and cream are all rich in calcium, vegans do not have the luxury of consuming them. Fortunately, there are alternatives. Many varieties of plant based vegan milk exists, but you must be sure to consume plant milk that is fortified with calcium AND vitamin D. Remember not to consume your calcium with legumes as the zinc and iron will bind to the calcium and inhibit the absorption by your body. Vitamin D is just as important as the calcium itself as it helps facilitate the absorption.

Choline is a lesser known essential nutrient, but healthy choline levels are critical to the function of your brain, nervous system, and liver[10]. While our body does produce choline naturally, you must derive more of it from food sources in order for your body to function properly. Tofu, cauliflower, and quinoa are all excellent sources of choline. If you enjoy drinking or are pregnant, your choline requirements are even higher and you should discuss your health needs with a doctor.

Who Could Forget Fruits and Vegetables

I know it seems insane to wait this long into the chapter, but fruits and vegetables are a cornerstone of the vegan diet. I think many vegans would agree the vast array of fruits and vegetables make the vegan diet manageable. Make no mistake, every piece of fresh produce is 100% vegan. It is only when you start eating prepared produce at restaurants do you run the risk of not eating vegan. Many restaurants now have vegan options to cater to a modern crowd. Fruits and vegetables are amazing as even eating them raw can make for a quick and easy snack. Almost any piece of fruit can be turned into a healthy, nutritious, vegan snack in just a minute. I would recommend to anyone attempting a vegan diet to have a wide array of fruits on hand for emergency snacking. Probably the most common pitfall on a diet is when you're hungry, busy, or both, and you don't know what to eat. Without a meal plan in place, you dive back into old habits and/or grab the first food in front of you. Hunger is a primal craving like thirst, sex, or checking your email. When your body is HONGRY, it's going to find food and take you along for the ride. The best way to avoid the HONGRIES is to have ready-to-go snacks you can munch on while you figure out a meal plan. Ideally, you always have a meal plan in place to avoid these situations, but we all know life doesn't work that way. You're busy, you forget, or dinner wasn't as filling as you thought it'd be, and suddenly you have cravings.

The easiest way to curb these cravings is to have some prepared fruit on hand ready to eat. Now I want to discuss a real danger of fruits and vegetables with you. Of course fruits and vegetables are insanely healthy for you, but more people actually get food poisoning from produce than from meat[11]. I know that sounds insane when you compare the dangers of undercooked meat to happy, healthy fruits and vegetables, but there's actually a very good reason for it. Most of the time, we don't cook our fruits and vegetables because we don't have to. I mean, how many times have you eaten a salad made from multiple uncooked vegetables? Or enjoyed a veggie platter? Or just grabbed an apple from the produce drawer? Cooking food kills bacteria, and that's why produce makes us so sick.

To combat food poisoning, the Center for Disease Control gives us a list of steps to minimize our exposure to dangerous bacteria found on produce[12].

1. At the store, always select produce that isn't bruised or damaged.
2. Always refrigerate prepared fruits and vegetables.
3. Always keep produce separate from raw meat.
4. Always wash your hands, utensils, and cutting surface before preparing fruits and vegetables.
5. Produce can be easily cleaned with just water and rubbing it with your clean hands.
6. Cut away any bruised or damaged portions of the produce.
7. Use a clean paper towel to dry the produce.
8. Cooking produce is an excellent way to make it safe for human consumption.
9. When preparing produce, refrigerate any unused portions within two hours at 40 degrees Fahrenheit.
10. When consuming sprouted vegetables, always consume them cooked whenever possible.
11. Children under 5 years of age, people over 65 years of age, and pregnant women are all at a higher risk for food poisoning.

Now that I've thoroughly ruined veganism for you, I want to talk about how amazing fruits and vegetables actually are. Remember, I'm here to give you the facts. I will never sugarcoat anything for you. Hiding the risks of raw produce would be entirely irresponsible of me. Despite those risks, fruits and vegetables are well worth it. Let's start with vegetables, and including fungus in here because it's just too darn *fun* to be left out of the party. *pauses for a mild chuckle*

If soy is the backbone of the vegan diet, then vegetables and fruit are the arms and legs. There are so many vegetables, and they're all so darn versatile you could go a whole year with veggie dishes and never eat the same thing twice. Hundreds of millions of Hindus spend their entire lives on a vegetarian diet, and you never hear them complain about all the delicious food they get to eat. One of my personal, favorite comfort foods is vegetable soup. Even the canned stuff is great. Whoa! Don't put the book down, let me explain first. Soup from a can is gross. Tastes like butt, and isn't really designed for anyone to enjoy. But if you've had a busy night writing a fantastic book, and you want a quick, satisfying meal, there's nothing like cracking open a canned of vegetable soup and relaxing. Now I know I just said canned soup is gross, that's because it is. But when you start adding your own vegetables to it, add some garlic, red pepper flakes, maybe some curry? Suddenly you have a taste explosion in your mouth. It takes a long time to stew vegetables, and you have to tend the stove and everything. Life is busy and it's only getting busier. I know I can take a can of veggie soup, spice it up, and have a satisfying meal with some vegan cheese and vegan crackers if I want to. There's just something about hot soup that makes your stomach happy.

Of course, it doesn't have to end at soup. Baby carrots and dressing are an awesome snack. Stir fried brocoli with garlic and black pepper is an awesome side dish. Salads are endless, especially when you combine them with nuts and fruits. Don't even get me started on eggplant! There are so many wonderful things you can do with vegetables. I just don't like how the media often portrays vegetables as these cold, tasteless punishments for children and fat people when vegetables are freakin' awesome! I could go an entire week just eating different veggie dishes and never get bored. And don't forget, vegetables create tons of interesting vegan substitutes. Pizza dough is vegan, but you can also have cauliflower pizza dough. You have veggie pasta and cauliflower mashed potatoes. Then you have mushrooms! Oh man, who could forget about mushrooms! They add such a delicious, umami flavor to any dish. You can grill them as burgers or add them to stir fries. They go great on pizza or a kebab. I know I sound like I'm gushing, but I want you to be as excited for veggies as I am. They're just so darn wonderful.

You have so many options. Salads, stir fries, vegan pizza, veggie lasagna, smoothies, veggie soup, casseroles. I could spend all day just naming vegetable treats. My point is, when you're excited about your food, it just makes the food taste better and feel more satisfying. You should get excited about what you eat. That's one of the joys of living. If you're bemoaning another veggie dish for dinner, you're either not being creative enough, or you might not be cut out for veganism. And that's okay if you don't feel you can be a vegan. But if there's one thing I want you to take away from all this, it's that you should get excited about what you eat. I promise it will improve the quality of your life.

And before we close this section, I think it's time we gushed a little about fruit. Now fruit is a difficult subject. While it's true that fruit is a tasty and delicious treat, it feels like more often than not when we buy fruit, it doesn't taste like it's supposed to. This isn't some strange phenomenon in your head, and especially in America, it can seem like fruits don't taste right just as often as they taste amazing. There is actually a reason for this, well a few actually[13]. For starters, Americans don't always purchase fruit when it's in season. Don't you think it's a little weird we have fresh fruit in the middle of January? Of course this fruit is shipped in from the southern hemisphere where our winter is their summer, but bear in mind there's only one harvest season. Since we consume basically all fruit all year-round, we're not always getting it at peak ripeness. Fruit is often picked before it's ready to harvest because chain grocery stores don't want holes in their stock. A place like Wal-Mart wants all apples for sale every day regardless if they are ready to be picked or not. This means you often end up biting into an unripe apple that isn't delicious or satisfying. You can eat a small delicious apple or a big bland apple, and I bet you feel more satisfied after the delicious one.

Another reason fruit feels like such a gamble is because American growers favor big, resilient produce over delicious produce[14]. Think about this, a farmer needs to sell so much food he or she grows in order to survive financially. There's a very good chance they sell to a distributor who handles many farmers. The distributor doesn't care what the food tastes like. Wal-Mart and Target both ordered so many tons of pickles (from pickle trees, of course) and they want them when they want them. The farmer isn't going to make more money selling delicious, farm raised pickles. The farmer is going to make money selling pickles that can survive insects, disease (the dreaded pickle syndrome), and maybe a light frost. If they are big bland pickles instead of tiny delicious pickles, then the farmer sells more tonnage of pickles and makes more money. It's quite the pickle when you think about it.

But there are ways to avoid these problems. To maximize your chances of delicious fruit, always buy in season. Below is a list of the most commonly purchased fruit and when you should purchase them[15].

- **Winter**: basically all varieties of oranges, bananas, avocados, kiwis, lemons, papayas, pomegranates, passion fruit, guava
- **Spring**: avocados, bananas, cherries, persimmons, pineapple, strawberries, oranges, papayas, passionfruit
- **Summer**: apricots, avocados, bananas, blackberries, blueberries, boysenberries, cantaloupe, cherries, figs, limes, mangoes, nectarines, oranges, papayas, passionfruit, peaches, plums, pineapples, raspberries, strawberries, watermelon
- **Winter**: apples, asian pears, avocados, bananas, clementines, cranberries, dates, grapes, guava, honeydew melon, kiwis, nectarines, oranges, papayas, passionfruit, plums, pomegranates, raspberries, strawberries, tangerines

Using this chart, you'll have much greater success with your fruit purchases. Another tactic is to only purchase produce at farmer's markets.

Farmer's markets generally only sell produce in season, but it's not unusual for a chain store to send their overstocked produce their to be sold. Talk to the farmers, get to know them. You'll quickly learn who is a legit farmer and
who is only there to sell overstocked fruits and vegetables. Not only will you receive better quality produce, but you'll also help small farmers make a living. At most farmer's markets, the cost is comparable to what you would pay at a chain store, but the money is going directly into the hands of the people who grew the food. It cuts away at the risk of mass contamination where hundreds of tons of produce are all transported together. Not only that, but there's a good chance you will meet other vegans at the market where you can swap stories and recipes. Even if you don't, I guarantee the farmer will have great suggestions on what to do with their produce since they're probably asked multiple times a day by customers.

The Ethics of Veganism

It is impossible to separate the vegan lifestyle from the ethics of veganism. In fact, the vast majority of vegans, more than 80%, cite concern for animals as their primary reason for going vegan[16]. When you objectively look at it, it's both inspiring and fascinating to undergo such a far reaching lifestyle change because of your ethical beliefs. This isn't as simple as ditching plastic water bottles or boycotting a corporation, this is a series of decisions a person undertakes every single day, at every single meal, in order to respect the life and value of animals. Regardless of your beliefs towards the food industry, you must admit that kind of action and determination is admirable. So few people back up their beliefs with their actions. As I said, it is relatively easy to boycott a restaurant for its political beliefs, or to stop buying straws, but in our western culture where 99.99% of restaurants serve meat as the primary menu options, it's astounding to watch vegans stay the course.

While it is admirable for a person to show such dedication to their beliefs, it is not admirable to force those beliefs on others. Remember, we can never know the complete circumstances of another person's life. As it turns out, high calorie junk food is much cheaper than nutrient rich produce. In a study by the USDA, they found that nutrient dense food can cost 10 times more per calorie than calorie dense food that is low in nutrients[17]. While fruits and vegetables may be cheaper per pound, it's not the amount of food we consume, but the amount of calories we need to survive. We don't know a person's life, and should never judge them for buying the food they need to survive. We don't all have an equal amount of opportunities, privileges, or resources, and those can drastically change where we end up in life. In fact, public activism is one of the least common ways people resort to veganism. Studies show that family and friends, followed by social media content, are the most common reasons people turn to veganism[20]. As it turns out, blogging and vlogging about veganism is one of the best ways to get people to join! I absolutely encourage you to talk to your friends and relatives about veganism without being condescending about it. I absolutely think it's a great idea if you want to start your own blog or Youtube channel where you discuss veganism and your own own personal experiences. Maybe tell them about the awesome vegan keto book you read? *Giant exaggerated wink*

I also want to take a moment and address the environmental sustainability of a vegan diet. You would be remiss to enter a vegan diet for environmental reasons, as a vegan diet is actually worse for the environment than a meat eating diet[18]. Now before you slam your tablet shut, allow me to explain. To quote the ground breaking study by Carnegie Mellon University[19],

"keeping calorie levels the same but adjusting the foods eaten to incorporate USDA recommendations that people eat more vegetables, fruits, dairy, and seafood would see energy use increase by 43 percent, with the water footprint increasing by 16 percent and emissions by 11 percent."

This may seem shocking and impossible, but when you look at the explanation, it actually makes a lot of sense. We know that beef and pork farms are filthy with tons of emissions and fecal run-off, but meat is extremely dense when it comes to calories. When you compare something like beef to brocoli, Beef has seven times the calories. And remember, we need calories to actually survive. It doesn't matter how many fruits and vegetables you eat if you're not meeting your daily minimum calories. I said many times before that I would not sugarcoat any of this for you. The facts are the facts. Eating vegan has a more negative environmental impact than eating meat. While it is truly admirable to want to protect the animals, eating vegan is not a proven way to protect the environment.

A Word About Raising Vegan Children

I would say that raising your children vegan is both one of the most controversial things you can do, and one of the most needlessly controversial things happening today. I'm going to put it bluntly and back it up with the facts. **It is absolutely safe and acceptable to raise your children vegan or vegetarian.** You don't even have to take my word for it, take the word of the American Academy of Pediatrics, British Dietetic Association, Academy of Nutrition and Dietetics, and Dietitians of Canada. In the Journal of the American Dietetic Association they write that a vegan and vegetarian diet is[20],

"appropriate for individuals during all stages of the lifecycle, including pregnancy, lactation, infancy, childhood, and adolescence, and for athletes."

And the Canadian Pediatric Society claims[21],

"well-planned vegetarian and vegan diets with appropriate attention to specific nutrient components can provide a healthy alternative lifestyle at all stages of fetal, infant, child and adolescent growth."

Yes, I intended to completely bury the argument when it comes to raising your children vegan or vegetarian. Despite what we see in the news where sick parents starve their children under the guise of a vegan diet, the fact of the matter is that when done properly under a doctor's care, veganism and vegetarianism is perfectly safe for children and infants. The news likes to sensationalize stories to draw attention, especially local news. I'm sure we've all seen a case or two where a parent or parents were starving their children and claiming they were vegans. The issue wasn't with what they were feeding their child, but how much they were feeding them. Veganism isn't child abuse. Starving your child is child abuse. I have personally worked in childcare before becoming a writer. You would have to willfully ignore hours and hours, days and weeks of crying and screaming to starve an infant or toddlers. It has nothing to do with veganism, and everything to do with sick people doing sick things.

Even though veganism and vegetarianism is perfectly safe and healthy for children and infants, special precautions must be taken. When raising your child as a vegan, it is extremely important that you do so under the supervision of a doctor. Infants especially require specific nutrients in order to develop properly. A vegan diet can be low in critical nutrients like protein, calcium, iron, and choline. The best way to avoid these issues is to breastfeed your child, but not every woman can breastfeed or wants to. In her book *Lactivism: How Feminists and Fundamentalists, Hippies and Yuppies, and Physicians and Politicians Made Breastfeeding Big Business and Bad Policy*, Courtney Jung flatly states that it takes the average woman 35 hours per week to breastfeed their child. Most women simply don't have that amount of free time, and if they do they often don't want to spend it feeding their child. The Academy of Nutrition and Dietetics recommends iron fortified soy formula if you do not or cannot breastfeed your child.

Even after they become toddlers and children, it is critical that you check in with your doctor regularly to make sure they are developing properly and are receiving all their vital nutrients. Your areas of nutritional focus should be iron, protein, calcium, vitamin D, and vitamin B12. Don't let anyone tell you that you can't raise your child vegan or vegetarian, even if it's your own doctor. If they say you have to make dietary changes, that's completely different than saying your child can't be vegan. Don't conflate the two and put your child at risk. The facts have been reiterated by every major institute and association that advises and monitors nutrition. If your doctor carries a prejudice against a vegan diet, you should seek out a new doctor. This isn't about righteousness or conflicting philosophies. Every major organization that studies nutrition says veganism and vegetarianism is safe for children and infants. One doctor doesn't know more about nutrition than the government bodies where people dedicate their lives to studying nutrition. It is easy to be intimidated by a doctor's authority or even be accused of child abuse because of the sensational stories in the news, but the facts are the facts.

In a world where more and more people handpick what they want to belief, it is more important than ever to know what the truth is. Remember earlier that I said I was arming you with knowledge. That knowledge will protect you from prejudice and willful ignorance. Don't be intimidated by others who disagree with your lifestyle. I wouldn't be saying these things if I hadn't researched the facts myself. If you want to be vegan and want your children to be vegan, it's no different from others eating meat and wanting their children to eat meat. Once your kids are adults, you can arm them with the knowledge of this book (makes a great gift) and they can decide for themselves if they want to continue to be vegan. The bottom line (too long, didn't read) is that you are not harming your child in any way by raising them as vegan or vegetarian.

What Makes Vegetarianism Different

And now to close the chapter with a section about vegetarianism. Vegetarianism and veganism are extremely similar diets and are often conflated when people discuss them. The only real difference between vegans and vegetarians is that vegetarians consume animal byproducts such as milk, eggs, and cheese while vegans abstain from animal products all together. I want you to know that everything we discussed about veganism applies to vegetarianism as well. All the dietary restrictions are in place, vegetarians should still buy their fruit seasonally for optimal taste, the politics of raising your child vegetarian can be just as difficult as raising them vegan, and the ethical implications of being vegetarian can be just as compelling as being vegan. Really, it all comes down to the difficulty of the diet. Veganism is not a lifestyle choice to be taken lightly. There are real restrictions involved. This goes doubly for a vegan keto diet. As stated previously, I don't want you to buy this book then feel like a failure because you couldn't stick to the difficult vegan keto diet. I want you to have options. My main goal is that you are completely satisfied with your purchase. That's why I dedicated an entire chapter just to vegetarian keto.

The main reason someone would choose to be vegetarian is ease of the diet and general nutrition. Since vegetarians are allowed to eat eggs, milk, and cheese, they can fill in a lot of the nutritional holes of the vegan diet. Milk and cheese are a good source of calcium and protein, eggs are loaded with protein and the critical B vitamins many vegans lack. There is no shame in being a vegetarian. It is still a proud and difficult lifestyle choice. I'd rather see you succeed as a vegetarian than fail as a vegan.

If vegetarianism isn't for you, there are actually many kinds of vegetarians who alter their diet to suit their needs. There are lacto-vegetarians who do not consume meat or eggs, but eat milk, cheese, yogurt, and other dairy products. This is a perfectly acceptable choice as milk and cheese make it very easy for you to get the necessary calcium and vitamin D your body needs to function. There are also ovo-vegetarians who do not eat meat or dairy products but consume eggs. The reasons for this are twofold. Many vegetarians want to avoid the hormones and antibiotics involved with the raising of cattle. Also, eggs are an excellent source of protein and B vitamins which are often absent from a vegetarian diet. There are also pollotarians who consume fowl but not red meat or fish. A pollotarian may or may not consume dairy and eggs. The twofold reason aside from the hormones and antibiotics in cattle is to also avoid the mercury involved with fish. A pollotarian focuses more on their health concerns than the ethical concerns a vegan might face as chicken is a very lean and healthy meat. Finally there are the pescatarians who are a branch of divinity that follow the teachings of the original Latin Church and claim to make an apostolic succession...wait a minute! That's Episcopalians! Pescatarians are a type of vegetarian who only consume fish as their source of meat. Like pollotarians, this is mainly for a reliable and healthy source of lean protein.

As you can see, there really is a diet for everyone. You can be as lose or as strict as you want to be. One of the great benefits of a vegetarian diet is that when done correctly, you are almost guaranteed to be healthier. I can attest from personal experience that amping up your fruit and vegetable consumption while cutting out beef and pork just makes you feel better. It's like your whole body functions better. Your brain, muscles, and digestion all seem to operate on a higher level when you practice being a vegetarian.

1.Wikipedia, *Veganism*, https://en.wikipedia.org/wiki/Veganism

2.The Vegan Society, *Definition of veganism*, https://www.vegansociety.com/go-vegan/definition-veganism

3. WedMD, *The Benefits of Protein*, Osterweil, Neil 2004 https://www.webmd.com/men/features/benefits-protein

4. Alternative Daily, *Tofu vs. Tempeh: There Is a Clear Winner* https://www.thealternativedaily.com/tofu-vs-tempeh/

5, 7, 8, 10. Healthline, *11 Foods Healthy Vegans Eat*, Petre, Alina, October 2016 https://www.healthline.com/nutrition/foods-vegans-eat

6. The Vegetarian Resource Group, *Iron in the Vegan Diet*, Mangels, Reed, PhD August 2018 https://www.vrg.org/nutrition/iron.php

9. Health.com, *The 15 Best Vegan Protein Powders*, Schlinger, Amy, January 2019 https://www.health.com/nutrition/best-vegan-protein-powder

11. Vox, *Fruits and vegetables poison more Americans than beef and chicken*, Belluz, Julia, March 2015 https://www.vox. com/2015/3/6/8158289/food-poisoning

12. CDC, *Fruit and Vegetable Safety*, https://www.cdc.gov/foodsafety/communication/steps-healthy-fruits-veggies.html

13, 14. Vox, *Why fruits and vegetables taste better in Europe*, Belluz, Julia, February 2016 https://www.vox.com/2016/2/12/10972140/fruits-vegetables-taste-better-europe

15. Shari's Berries, *What Fruits Are In Season? Easy Reference Chart*, Daniels, Erica, March 2017 https://www.berries.com/blog/what- fruits-are-in-season

16. Vomad Life, *Why Most People Go Vegan: 2016 Survey Results Revealed*, Hersham M December 2016 https://vomadlife.   com/blogs/news/why-most-people-go-vegan-2016-survey-results-reveal-all

17. The Simple Dollar, *Low Calorie Food and Longterm Costs*, Hamm, Trent, August 2014 https://www.thesimpledollar.com/low-calorie-food-and-long-term-costs/

18, 19. Science Alert, *Vegetarian And 'Healthy' Diets May Actually Be Worse For The Environment*, Study Finds, Dockrill, Peter, December https://www.sciencealert.com/vegetarian-and-healthy-diets-may-actually-be-worse-for-the-environment-study-finds

20. Journal of the American Dietetic Association, *Position of the American Dietetic Association: Vegetarian Diets*, July 2009 https://jandonline.org/article/S0002-8223%2809%2900700-7/fulltext

Why Vegan Keto?

As you know by now, the vegan keto diet is one of the most difficult and restrictive diets you can go on. A lot of the most reliable vegan foods such as every fruit imaginable except for avocados and coconuts are off the table when you combine a vegan diet with a keto diet. Protein is more difficult to come by as all beans are off the table as well. Beans are very high in carbs compared to the amount of protein they provide. Even eating excess protein will stop your body from entering ketosis as it will convert any excess protein it doesn't need into glucose. Tofu is not a great substitute either as consuming large amounts of unfermented, processed soy contains numerous health risks. If you recall earlier I mentioned that soy contains high levels of phytates. These antioxidants act as antinutrients and hormones and interfere greatly with the natural processes of your body. Phytates can bind to the nutrients in your food and prevent your body from absorbing them[1]. Some phytates are known as phyto-estrogen and literally raise the estrogen levels in your body causing infertility and elevated risks of cancer in women, and decreased sex drive and breasts in men (known as gynecomastia)[2]. And on to top it all off, you can't eat starchy vegetables because they're loaded with carbs. This includes potatoes, sweet potatoes, yams, pumpkin, squash, or peas.

Because of the health risks associated with the excess consumption of tofu, it is advised you consume tempeh and natto as a replacement, as the fermentation process breaks down the dangerous phytates in the soy. In the following chapters, we will suggest other food replacements and even give you a two week diet plan to help you stick with a vegan keto diet.

It's easy to see why a vegan keto diet is so challenging. Not only are reliable vegan staples tossed out the window, but you must also be sure to induce ketosis or the entire diet is useless. Even if you do eat all the correct foods, if you eat them in the wrong proportions, then the diet doesn't even work. Bear in mind ketosis is a scientifically proven phenomenon where your body stops using glucose for food and turns to ketones instead. This only happens when you reduce your carbohydrate consumption to just 5% of your total calories. If you can't follow the 5% rule, then the diet is completely useless. So why would anyone want to follow a vegan keto diet?

Ethics

There is almost no research done on the combination of veganism and keto, but I would bet the main reason you would want a vegan version of the keto diet is because of your ethical concerns for animals. We already learned that over 80% of vegans cite concern for animals as their main reason for going vegan[3]. I really want to reiterate that this is a very admirable reason to choose veganism. Your concern for animals is so great you would forsake a vast portion of the western diet just to protect them. It cannot be overstated that in a world where so few people actually act on their convictions, you choose everyday and at every meal to put your concern for animals over the luxury of many readily available foods. That's admirable.

It's great you want to carry your concern for all living creatures all the way through the restrictive keto diet. Keto has many, many health benefits including reduced risk of obesity and heart disease, better gut health, and higher energy levels[4]. When you combine the amazing health benefits with the vegan ethical philosophy, it may seem like we have discovered the most perfect diet of all time. Well that may be debatable, I'm not writing this book to argue against how amazing this diet is. But I would be remiss if I didn't reiterate the challenges of the vegan keto diet. The food selection is extremely restrictive and most restaurants won't be able to accommodate you. If you don't follow the 5% rule, you won't receive any of the health benefits of a keto diet. But this all makes sense if you take a moment to think about it. If a diet has so many incredible health benefits and also respects all living creatures, then surely it would be difficult. If it was easy, everyone would do it.

The best things in life are challenging. So many people behave unethically because it's easy. It's almost always difficult to do the right thing. Why work for 40 hours to buy a new TV when you could just steal one? If you found a wallet with a thousand dollars in it, it would be very easy to keep the money. It's not like you even really stole it, you found it. But it's much more difficult to return that money without any expectation of a reward. It's easy, affordable, and accessible to find and eat junk food. Junk food is cheap, satisfying, everywhere, and everyone already eats it. But for your longterm health, it's better to never touch the stuff. Many people find meat delicious. The taste, the smell, the protein and energy it gives. But there is no doubt the vast majority of animals live short and miserable lives just to be turned into food. Our entire food culture in the west is based around the consumption of animals. You would be hard pressed to find a single restaurant that doesn't serve meat. Even if you go to an ice cream shop, there's a strong chance they serve hotdogs, pizza, and/or nachos. Even movie theaters sell that stuff! You can go to a salad place and they'll still serve you salad with chicken or anchovies on it. Meat is everywhere. Make no mistake, it is difficult in western civilization to live a life where you don't consume meat.

Only .5% of Americans are vegan[5]. That's not a lot of people, and western civilization isn't really set up to meet the needs of vegan people. Also remember vegans choose to be vegan. This isn't something you're born as like being black or transgender. This is an active choice you make. A choice you have to reinforce everyday at every snack and every meal. It is a massive ethical choice that shapes your entire life, one that is difficult to stick to. Remember, it's not supposed to be easy. The ethical choices are almost never easy.

Knowledge

Knowledge is another excellent reason to choose a vegan keto diet. The fact of the matter is, a lot is known about veganism including its history, diet, benefits, and health risks. The same can be said for keto. We know the risks and the benefits. We know the exact process in the body that causes ketosis and subsequently causes an inspiring amount of weight loss. But there is very limited information about combining the two into an effective diet. I've gathered every single piece of information I could find about keto and veganism and condensed them down into this book with full citations and references so what I say is always backed up by fact. You can do your own research as well. I want this to be the go-to book for anyone considering a vegan keto diet. I truly believe *Vegan Keto* is a font of knowledge where anyone can learn all they ever wanted to know about keto, veganism, vegetarianism, standard keto, vegetarian keto, and the glorious vegan keto diet.

But remember, our search is never ending. I truly believe one of our goals as human beings is to gather as much knowledge as possible, not just from the world around us, but from ourselves as well. I want this book to be the handbook of vegan keto diets, but I also want you to continue your quest for knowledge. I do not have the kind of hubris to say this is the only source of vegan keto knowledge you will ever need. I would never say to ignore everyone else who writes about vegan keto. We all bring different things to the table. No source of information is perfect. You are on a journey of food and diet knowledge. You are privy to a way of food life that few will ever know. Never stop learning. Go to the sources I cited and learn everything you can about veganism, ketogenics, and how the two combine to form a powerful diet. Discuss your knowledge with others. Talk about it on social media. Blog about it. The world is so vast. I genuinely believe that our human world contains an infinite number of facets for us to discover.

This isn't just about a diet. This is a chance for you to learn everything you can about veganism. I want you to learn about the treatment of animals on meat farms, but I also want you to learn about the treatment of migrant workers who harvest your food. I want you to learn about the environmental impact of corporate meat farms, but I also want you to learn about the greater impact growing produce has on the environment. Yes, it's true. Growing produce has a more negative impact on the environment than raising animals for food[6]. But I don't want you to take my word for it, nor do I want you to blindly disagree with me. I want you to go to the work I cited and do your own research.

That's what's so great about these two diets combining to form a super diet. Veganism forces you to question where your food comes from, how it's grown, and how it gets to your plate. I feel these are questions the average American rarely considers. Keto forces you to learn there are other ways of eating, and there are diets that actually work. Forever, biologists knew that our body is fueled by glucose. This was generally accepted, scientific fact. What else could your body possibly run on? Well as it turns out, your body can run on ketones with a proper diet. Not only is glucose unnecessary for your body to function, but according to all preliminary evidence, it runs pretty darn good on ketones. Through the information just like the kind found in this book, we are literally questioning everything we knew about the human body. Forever, scientists said your body needs meat in order to function. But that quaint notion has been destroyed a thousand times over by millions of people who live completely healthy lives free from animal products.

When you think about it, we're really like food pioneers traveling into the great unknown. There is such limited information about a vegan keto diet, we're basically like the first team of explorers charting a brand new land. Vegan keto is a brave new world for us to explore. It could be the secret to a long life, fighting cancer, or treating chronic inflammation which is the underlying cause of so many debilitating diseases. I don't want you to keep this book as some special secret. I want you to tell everyone about this book. For one, it'll make me all the money, but just as importantly, it will give us allies in this diet adventure. I want you to blog about it. I want you to write articles about it. I want you to go on Youtube and talk about your vegan keto experiences both good and bad. It is human nature to explore the unknown. You don't even have to leave your town or city to undergo this great expedition.

If you can get excited and passionate about your new diet, then you're that much more likely to stick with it. I want you to love this. I want you to hate this. Most importantly, I want you to have strong feelings about vegan keto. I am relaying to you every piece of information I know and can find about vegan keto, but there's so much more we don't know. What are the longterm effects of a vegan keto diet? What are the unknown health benefits of a vegan keto diet? What obscure foods can we bring into the mainstream with a vegan keto diet? I don't have the resources to answer these questions. But if we can create awareness and buzz for vegan keto, if we can get people as excited as we are, it will only be a matter of time before we find some answers.

Life Saving Benefits

After the ethical implications of veganism, I feel the second most common reason a person would choose a vegan keto diet is for the numerous health benefits. There are many preliminary studies that illustrate a correlation between keto and powerful health benefits. Remember, correlation is not causation, but it's exciting to discover the possible health benefits of your body burning ketones instead of glucose.

Fighting heart disease may be one of the most vital reasons to undergo a vegan keto diet. The Center for Disease control estimates that heart disease kills 610,000 Americans every year. That means that when you take into account every single death in the entire country, 1 out of every 4 deaths is caused by heart disease[7]. That is absolute insanity. That also means that heart disease is the number one cause of death for black people, white people, and Hispanic people[8]. It's hard to imagine one thing can kill so many people, but the numbers don't lie. Again, I never want you to simply accept what I say at face value. Do your own research and get informed. I think you'll discover there is a lot of evidence a keto diet reduces your risk of heart disease[9]. Through my own personal research, I've found strong evidence for why keto is such a good diet for your heart health. You would think a high fat diet would wreck havoc on your heart, but it's actually your blood glucose levels that damage the function of your heart. High levels of blood glucose damages our blood vessels which is why diabetes is so closely associated with cardiovascular problems. High blood sugar also damages the nerves that control our heart[10]. This isn't some scare tactic a keto guru came up with to drive page views, this information comes directly from the National Institute of Diabetes and Digestive and Kidney Diseases, and I'm pretty sure they know what they're talking about.

I know I sound like I'm talking about some kind of magic wonder diet, but studies suggest keto may also be used to treat cancer as well[11]. In 2018, over 1.7 million Americans were diagnosed with cancer, and over 609,000 people died from cancer that same year. That makes cancer the second leading cause of death only behind heart disease[12]. Cancer is a miserable, heartless disease that destroys so many lives. While treatments are limited, some studies suggest keto could be a new treatment in the future. Let me be absolutely frank; vegan keto will not cure your cancer or cure the cancer of a loved one. Keto can only be used as a TREATMENT for cancer, and only certain kinds of cancer at that. Always consult with a doctor before changing your diet, especially if you have a medically recommended diet for your cancer treatment.

Though there are few studies on the treatment of cancer with keto, the ones that have been published show mindblowing results. On a study of mice with cancer, scientists found mice that were fed a keto diet had a 60% survival rate compared to a 0% survival rate for mice on a normal diet. When the study was replicated by combining a ketogenic diet with ketone supplements, the survival rate of the keto mice increased to 100%[13]! Those are mindblowing results to say the least. Unfortunately, the research into the cancer treatment in humans is very limited. While multiple studies and cases have shown a positive link between keto diet and cancer survival rate[14], none of them are scientifically conclusive enough to definitively prove keto is an effective cancer treatment. Basically what we're stuck with is small study after small study after small study that shows a beneficial link between keto and cancer treatment, but no single study large enough to draw conclusions.

There are even known scientific mechanisms in place that would explain why keto is such an effective cancer treatment. Scientists know cancer cells use glucose as energy just like every other cell in our body. We also know people who have difficulty managing their blood sugar are at an increase risk of cancer[14]. But what happens when you don't have blood sugar? What happens when your body uses ketones for energy instead of glucose? All available information suggests cancer really doesn't like that. A wide variety of studies suggest a keto diet inhibits the growth of tumors, and when people end their keto diet, the tumors resume a more traditional rate of growth. The limited information available would seem to suggest a strict keto diet can starve cancer. Remember, your doctor went to school for 11 years, and probably even more if they're an oncologist. You need to take their professional medical advice over mine. But, and this is a big but, I cannot lie, you can absolutely bring this book to your doctor. You can print out the references and studies I have cited for you. Cancer is a f*cking scumbag. Cancer is a war. My mom beat cancer twice, and I wouldn't wish it on my worst enemies. You deserve every available weapon in your battle for cancer. If your oncologist refuses to even read the material, you might need to ask for a new one. This is not about taking my advice over a professional's, this is about having all the information available to you. This is about having every weapon at hand in order to fight cancer. If you are in the fight of your life, then I wish you the best of luck. There is always something you can do, some way to fight. There are no guarantees in life, but if you want to fight this evil thing, don't let anyone stop you.

Weight Loss

To begin, I would like to point out the main reason people go on a keto diet is weight loss, not necessarily why people go on a vegan keto diet. Either way, when done correctly, you are guaranteed to lose weight no matter how much food you eat. When you combine real weight loss with unlimited snacking, then it's easy to see why the keto diet is so popular. I'm about to lay some shocking numbers on you, so you may want to sit down. As of 2016, the most recent years reliable statistics are available, 71.6% of Americans are overweight(including obese people), and 39.8% of Americans are obese[15]. That means that 39.8% of Americans are obese, 31.8% of Americans are overweight but not obese, and 28.4% of Americans are normal weight or less. That's really messed up. No one really knows why Americans are so fat now, but everyone thinks they do. Like all massive phenomenons, the causes are many.

Through my personal research, I've found many studies and theories about why we are so fat today. First I want to discuss the misconceptions surrounding hormones and antibiotics given to animals. The two are often conflated as we search for a cause to the obesity epidemic, but only one of them has been tested to show it contributes to weight gain. Despite what we read in the news, hormones given to cattle are not making us fatter. When you look at the hard numbers, you'll find it's actually impossible for the hormones in beef to make us fatter. Agricultural economist Jayson Lusk has written an eye opening article about the fake hormone epidemic which I've cited for you. As it turns out, hormone treated beef has 7 nanograms of estrogen hormones per serving, while hormone free beef only has 5 nanograms per 500 gram serving[16]. At first that might seem massive. You don't need a lot of hormones to have a huge impact on the body. Going from 5 to 7 nanograms is a 40% increase. But then you start comparing it to other foods, and you see why there is no possible way beef hormones are having any effect on your health. Simple white bread you buy in the grocery store has 300,000 nanograms per 500 gram serving, pinto beans have a whopping 900,000 nanograms per serving, and tofu has an earth shatter 113 million nanograms of estrogen hormones per serving[17]! Do you see why it is impossible for beef hormones to have any effect on your health whatsoever? Eating just a slice of plain bread is the same as 40,000 servings of beef when it comes to hormones.

Antibiotics on the other hand are a completely different story. The reason antibiotics have such a negative affect on your weight is because they kill, or sometimes strengthen, certain bacteria in your gut. While it's hard to count them all, scientists believe you may have up to two pounds of solid bacteria living in your intestines at any given time. These bacteria do a ton of things including converting calories from one form to another, absorbing calories, and absorbing the water you need to live. Antibiotics cause the antibodies in your bod to wake up and start killing all the bacteria. It's basically the ultimate ding-dong-ditch. Bacteria are screwing around in your front yard, making you sick, and antibiotics run up and push the door bell, making your antibodies realize there's a bunch of no good bacteria on the lawn. Unfortunately, your antibodies can't tell deadly bacterial infections from the helpful flora that lives in your tummy. Generally when a doctor prescribes us an antibiotic, our antibodies wake up, we might have some crappy side effects, but then eventually everything goes back to normal. But when antibodies are in our food, we're under a constant, daily low dose of antibiotics that fundamentally change the bacteria neighborhood in our gut. The micro-dosing of antibiotics from food can kill certain bacteria making problematic ones grow stronger. Some bacteria are really efficient at absorbing calories for your body. Other bacteria turn carbohydrates into fatty acids, which eventually become lipids(fat) in your body. I'm citing two articles for you to review at your leisure after the book, but the gist is, study after study has found a link to the micro-doses of hormones found in beef, to obesity and fat retention[18,19].

Other scientists purport that we lead less active lives, consume more calories, and the advent of central air means our body doesn't have to work as hard to keep us warm in winter and cool in the summer. The fact of the matter is we are fatter than at any time in history. For the first time in history, this generation of children is expected to have a shorter life expectancy than their parents[20], and keto may be the solution to it all. That's right, if trends continue as they are now, our children will live shorter, unhealthier lives than we did. That's really sad to think the obesity epidemic has gotten this bad. But keto can really be the answer. I'm citing an article with over 15 different studies that suggest keto is an extremely effective weight loss plan[21]. The facts and evidence are there. You have the meal plans and guidelines in front of you. Now it's all about getting out there and taking the necessary actions to lose weight. Weight loss is absolutely possible. I know it sounds like some impossibility to radically change your physical makeup, but it is possible. I don't care if you ultimately choose the vegan keto diet, the vegetarian keto diet, or the standard keto diet. I just want you to end up in a place in your life where you are happier and healthier. Yes this book is going to make me money, but it's also a ton of work. Look at how much freakin' research I did in the notes! I really do want you to get healthier. That makes this work so immensely satisfying, knowing that this book could actually help people live better lives. It gives me a purpose. Helping you is my purpose. I want your purpose to be helping yourself.

Diabetes

At this point it might seem like keto is some outerspace diet given to us by aliens. How could such a simple diet do so much for our health? It can prevent heart disease, be used as a cancer treatment, and even end obesity. But what if it could do more? What if it could treat diabetes? Yes, diabetes. According to the Center for Disease Control, 30.3 million Americans have diabetes, and another 84.1 are pre-diabetic meaning if they don't change their lifestyle or begin medication they will develop diabetes within 5 years[22]. Those are some startling numbers. But as it turns out, preliminary studies have shown the keto diet is an excellent treatment for diabetes and a lack of insulin sensitivity. The diabetes we are talking about specifically is type 2 diabetes where your body produces too much insulin because it has lost sensitivity to it. In one study, scientists found that the keto diet increases your sensitivity to insulin by a whopping 75%[23]. Losing weight can also help you manage your diabetes, and we already know keto is excellent at helping people lose weight.

Remember, the keto diet induces ketosis in your body. Ketosis means your body stops using glucose and starts using ketones for energy. Without blood sugar, you no longer have to worry about insulin sensitivity. Insulin tells your body how to use blood sugar and when and where to store it. But if your body is operating on ketones, you no longer need to produce insulin as your blood sugar is gone.

Neurological Diseases

Finally, the last health benefit we will cover is the disease the ketogenic diet was originally designed for. Back at the turn of the century, the ketogenic diet was created to help children manage their epileptic seizures. The diet actually disappeared shortly after as effective anticonvulsants soon entered the market. But now that interest in keto has sparked again, we have learned that not only is it great at reducing seizures in people with epilepsy, but it could also be an effective treatment for debilitating neurological diseases like Alzheimer's and Parkinson's[24]. While no one is claiming that keto will cure Alzheimer's, epilepsy, or Parkinson's, there is strong evidence cited that a keto diet can greatly help to manage symptoms.

There are two working theories about why keto is such an effective treatment for neurological disorders. First, we learned in the heart disease sectio blood sugar can cause damage to blood vessels and the nervous system, especially at elevated levels. This isn't exclusive to the heart and may in fact damage nerves and blood vessels in the brain. With a keto diet removing all your blood sugar, scientists theorize it gives your body a break from slow, accumulating damage and allows itself to heal.

The other theory is certain neurological disorders are caused because your brain isn't receiving enough calories, effectively short circuiting it. But remember, keto burns massive amount of calories, and that includes calories burned by your brain. Our brain accounts for 20% of our calorie needs, burning hundreds of calories a day just to function[25]. Scientists theorize when our brain doesn't receive enough calories, it causes parts to die or degenerate. Fortunately for us, keto is like a calories furnace and the ketones provide all the energy our brains need.

1, 2. Alternative Daily, *Tofu vs. Tempeh: There Is a Clear Winner* https://www.thealternativedaily.com/tofu-vs-tempeh/

3. Vomad Life, *Why Most People Go Vegan: 2016 Survey Results Revealed*, Hersham M December 2016 https://vomadlife.   com/blogs/news/why-most-people-go-vegan-2016-survey-results-reveal-all

4. Dr. Jockers, *How to Follow a Vegan Ketogenic Diet*, Dr. Jockers https://drjockers.com/follow-vegan-ketogenic-diet/

5. Vegan Bits, *VEGAN DEMOGRAPHICS 2017 – USA, AND THE WORLD*, 2017 http://veganbits.com/vegan-demographics-2017/

6. Science Alert, *Vegetarian And 'Healthy' Diets May Actually Be Worse For The Environment*, Study Finds, Dockrill, Peter,   December https://www.sciencealert.com/vegetarian-and-healthy-diets-may-actually-be-worse-for-the-environment-study-finds

7, 8. Center for Disease Control, *Heart Disease Facts*, February 2015 https://www.cdc.gov/heartdisease/facts.htm

,9 21, 23, 24. Healthline, *The Ketogenic Diet: A Detailed Beginner's Guide to Keto*, Mawer, Rudy, July 2018, https://www. healthline. com/nutrition/ketogenic-diet-101

10. National Institute of Diabetes and Digestive and Kidney Diseases, *Diabetes, Heart Disease, and Stroke* Buse, John B. M.D. Ph.D. https://www.niddk.nih.gov/health-information/diabetes/overview/preventing-problems/heart-disease-stroke

11. Healthline, *Can the Keto Diet Help Fight Cancer?* Fischer, Kristen October 2018 https://www.healthline.com/health-news/can-the-keto-diet-help-fight-cancer

12. National Cancer Institute, *Cancer Statistics*, April 2018 https://www.cancer.gov/about-cancer/understanding/statistics

13. Healthline, *Can a Ketogenic Diet Help Fight Cancer?*, Mawer, Rudy, July 2016 https://www.healthline.com/nutrition/ketogenic-diet-to-fight-cancer

14. WedMD, *Why Does Diabetes Raise Cancer Risk?*, DeNoon, Daniel J., July 2010 https://www.webmd.com/diabetes/news/20100616/why-does-diabetes-increase-cancer-risk

15, 20. Center for Disease Control and Prevention, *Obesity and Overweight*, May 2017 https://www.cdc.gov/nchs/fastats/obesity-overweight.htm

16, 17. jaysonlusk.com, *Hormones in Soybeans and Beef*, Lusk, Jayson, July 2014 http://jaysonlusk.com/blog/2014/7/14/hormones-in-soybeans-and-beef

18. Scientific American, *Antibiotics Linked to Weight Gain*, Maxmen, Army, August 2012 https://www.scientificamerican. com/article/antibiotics-linked-weight-gain-mice/

19. University of California Berkeley, *Are Antibiotics Making us Fat?*, April 2015 http://www.berkeleywellness.com/healthy-eating/food/food-safety/article/are-antibiotics-food-making-people-fat

. The New York Times, *Children's Life Expectancy Being Cut Short by Obesity*, Belluck, Pam, March 2005 https://www.nytimes. com/2005/03/17/health/childrens-life-expectancy-being-cut-short-by-obesity.html

. Center for Disease Control, *New CDC report: More than 100 million Americans have diabetes or prediabetes*, July 2017 https://www.cdc.gov/media/releases/2017/p0718-diabetes-report.html

. Scientific American, Does Thinking Really Hard Burn More Calories?, Jabr, Ferris, July 2012 https://www.scientificamerican. com/article/thinking-hard-calories/

Side Effects of a Keto Diet

While the keto diet really seems like a miracle diet, there is no such thing as the perfect diet. Every diet contains health risks, even keto. Some of them are very mild, while others can be life threatening. It would be morally irresponsible of me to talk about the keto diet and recommend it to others without discussing the risks associated with ketosis. I strongly urge you to speak with a doctor about your diet plans before making any major changes.

Keto Flu

One of the most common side effects you might hear about associated with keto is what is know colloquially as "keto flu". This is not a viral infection like influenza, but instead a grouping of flu-like symptoms many people experience in the first days of ketosis. These symptoms are caused by your body adapting to the ketones in your blood stream, while others are actually symptoms of other symptoms. Symptoms of keto flu include, but are not limited to[1]:

- Vomiting
- Constipation
- Diarrhea
- Headache
- Irritability
- Weakness
- Muscle cramps
- Dizziness
- Poor concentration
- Stomach pain
- Muscle soreness
- Difficulty sleeping
- Sugar cravings
- Nausea

I know that sounds like a lot of side effects, but you are most likely only going to experience a few of them, and only for less than a week. Many of those symptoms are caused by dehydration. When you are in ketosis, your body starts to burn up your fat stores. Your body stores water in all that fat and can no longer rely on it. You may also find yourself urinating a lot. Almost all of those symptoms can be relieved just by staying well hydrated during your diet, which is just sound advice in general.

It is also recommended you do not do any strenuous exercises as your body adapts to the ketones in your blood stream. Strenuous exercise can also compound problems with dehydration and lost electrolytes, so it's best to avoid it in the first week. Keto is such a powerful diet you don't actually need to exercise to lose weight. If you are doing keto to manage your weight, 80% of the amount of weight you lose is attributed to your diet[2]. There's no reason you have to tear it up in the gym to lose weight on keto, especially your first week.

Avoiding caffeine is also a good strategy. People usually aren't prepared for the massive blast of energy they'll receive when they enter ketosis. Remember, your body is burning so much energy that if you ate bacon and butter at every meal you'd still lose weight. That's how much your metabolism will increase on the keto diet. There's a very good chance you won't need caffeinated beverages to function anymore. When you combine caffeine with the energy of a keto diet, you can find it difficult to fall asleep or concentrate. It's best just to avoid caffeine all together or at the very least in the first couple weeks of keto.

Keep in mind keto flu doesn't affect everyone, but it also affects people in different ways. It can actually be a good sign you're experiencing keto flu. That means your body is actually entering ketosis and you're doing the diet correctly. Most symptoms don't last longer than a week, and again most symptoms can be relieved with just a few simple beverage choices and a good night's sleep. If symptoms last longer than a week, I urge you to make an appointment with your doctor.

Keto Breath

The second most common side effect of keto is what is known as "keto breath". Keto breath is not just limited to your breath but can also make your urine, sweat, and your vagina smell funny. Though it might seem like a mental thing, there is actually a clear reason why keto would cause your bodily secretions to smell strange. Remember, ketosis is when your body starts using ketones for energy instead of glucose. While some ketones are used primarily for energy, your liver makes other ketones as a result of the process. One of those ketones is acetate. You might know it as acetone or nail polish remover. That's right, your body is literally pumping out nail polish remover during ketosis. It's not really toxic at all, but it can make your bodily fluids smell like nail polish remover. This doesn't affect everyone who does keto, but can be an annoying, if temporary side effect. The best remedy is to just drink plenty of water. While this is no guarantee for eliminating keto breath or what they call "keto crotch", it can help you manage your symptoms.

Ketoacidosis

Ketoacidosis is a condition where too much ketones exist in your blood stream making it so acidic that it kills you. Now before you toss the book across the room, you should know that ketoacidosis is incredibly rare and usually only affects people with type 1 diabetes without them even being on a keto diet. Because of this, I would never recommend anyone with type 1 diabetes to attempt a keto diet. If you insist on trying the keto diet, only do so under strict supervision from your doctor. Ketoacidosis is an extremely dangerous blood condition that can kill you very painfully.

If you are not type 1 diabetic, then there isn't really a threat of keto acidosis. The level of ketones in your urine (how they generally measure this) is less than .6millimol/liter. Above that, you are entering ketosis. You have to go all the way up to 10millimol/liter to experience ketoacidosis[3]. That's nearly twenty times the levels of ketones in your body!

Ketoacidosis is a very cornercase side effect of the keto diet that won't really effect you unless you have type 1 diabetes, but I believe it is important to illuminate all the risks of the diet, so you can make an educated decision about your body.

1. Healthline, *The Keto Flu: Symptoms and How to Get Rid of It*, Kubala, Jillian, April 2018, https://www.healthline.com/nutrition/keto-flu-symptoms
2. Center for Nutritional Studies, *Healthy Weight Loss = 80% Nutrition + 20% Exercise*, Edwards, Terri January 2018 https://nutritionstudies.org/healthy-weight-loss-80-nutrition-20-exercise/
3. Healthline, *Ketosis vs. Ketoacidosis: What You Should Know*, Butler, Natalie, February 2018 https://www.healthline.com/health/ketosis-vs-ketoacidosis

The Vegan Keto Diet

Here it is! What you've been waiting for this entire time. I bet there's a good chance you just skipped to this chapter first. I strongly urge you to go back and learn all the valuable information surrounding the ketogenic diet and veganism, especially the health risks associated with both diets. But I'm not your mother, so I can't stop you. Without further ado, I'm going to introduce you to the principles and practices of a vegan keto diet. At the end of the book will be a two week meal plan you can follow or tweak to your own preferences. The meal plan isn't set in stone. You can swap meals around or close your eyes and point at a random one if you're feeling whimsical.

The most core principle of the keto diet is that only 5% of your calories are allowed to come from carbs. It seems very simple, but there is no bend or give to this rule. If you do not restrict your carbohydrate intake to 5%, then you won't enter ketosis, and you won't receive any of the benefits of ketogenic diet. It really is that simple.

On top of that, only 20% of your calories can come from protein. Now this number is a little more flexible as active people require higher amounts of protein than sedentary people. Protein intake can go as high as 35% of total calories, but that is only really for athletes. If you consume too many calories from protein, your body turns the excess protein into glucose, and then you never enter ketosis.

On the standard diet, this means 75% of all calories you consume must come from fats. On a vegan diet, that is very difficult. Vegans are not allowed to eat cream, cheese, or eggs which are three staple foods on the vegetarian and standard keto diet. There are other options, but those options are limited.

Because a high fat diet is critical to inducing ketosis, your vegan keto diet will be based around avocados, olives, coconut products, and high fat nuts such as macadamia nuts. That's not to say you're going to be eating sliced avocado and olives out of half a coconut everyday, but they will be daily staples of your diet. Remember, the more fat calories you consume, the more room you have for protein and carb calories. Keto does not restrict the amount of calories you can eat, it only places restrictions on the ratio of calories you can eat. If you eat a ton of fatty plants and plant products, then you can eat other foods too.

Protein isn't critical to a keto diet as it is usually ingested incidentally with high fat foods, but when we talk about the vegan aspect of a vegan keto diet, then you absolutely must take into account your protein intake. I know vegans love their tofu, but it's not exactly healthy to be eating unfermented soy everyday. In the vegan section we talked about the dangers of phytates in soy which can cause numerous health problems and even bind to the nutrients in food, preventing your body from absorbing them. Fermented soy products like tempeh and natto beans are safe to consume daily because the fermentation process breaks down the phytates.

Aside from those considerations, I also recommend incorporating lots and lots of mushrooms into your vegan keto diet. The vegan keto diet can feel so restrictive, and you shouldn't be eating tofu every day, so mushrooms are a great alternative. They have so many uses including salads, stir fries, and veggie pastas. You can grill them or just fry them in oil with spices and garlic. Trust me when I say you always want a variety of mushrooms on hand when you do vegan keto as they're just so versatile and easy to create a meal with.

As a snack, there are many keto chips[1] and keto crackers[2] available, but you can also make your own. When eating these chips and crackers, guacamole makes the perfect vegan keto dip because of the high fat content. Remember, the more fat you eat, the less likely you'll be to go over your carb limit. Walnuts and macadamia nuts are also a great snack to have on hand. Even salted and roasted, they're the perfect food to grab and munch with no preparation needed. Because of the indulgent nature of the keto diet, there should rarely be a time that you're hungry. But sometimes you just get a craving. It's super important to have these salty, crispy snacks on hand so you can battle a craving with the exact taste and texture you're craving.

If you're craving something sweet, whole fat coconut milk can be used in a ton of dishes to make sweet treats with stevia. Remember that keto is based on your calorie ratios, not your total calories, so when making something yummy like lemon cookie bites[3], or keto ice cream[4], you're allowed to incorporate small bits of fruit.

This is all I can teach you without getting into the specifics of a meal plan. The vegan keto diet is absolutely doable, and I think you will learn a lot about yourself and the world of food in the process. You are combining a powerful diet with many known health benefits with an ethical food philosophy. Expect many changes if you can stay the course. If you find yourself struggling to stick to a vegan keto diet, that's perfectly fine. Not everyone is cut out for such a restrictive diet. No one's perfect. You can still enjoy an ethical food philosophy and powerful health benefits under the vegetarian keto diet. Going vegetarian opens you up to cheese and eggs which create numerous and exciting meal options. You are not a failure because you failed at one of the most challenging diets ever. Failing is how we learn about ourselves. The important thing is you tried to make it work. There are other options out there for you. I know if you stick with it, you'll find a diet plan that satisfies you. Just never give up.

1. Dr. Jockers, *Crunchy Garlic Keto Chips*, Dr. Jockers, https://drjockers.com/garlic-keto-chips/
2. Dr. Jockers, *Homemade Keto Crackers*, Dr. Jockers, https://drjockers.com/homemade-keto-crackers/
3. Dr. Jockers, *Coconut Lemon Glazed Cookie Bites*, Dr. Jockers, https://drjockers.com/coconut-lemon-glazed-cookie-bites/
4. Dr. Jockers, *Berry Coconut Milk Ice Cream*, Dr. Jockers, https://drjockers.com/berry-coconut-milk-ice-cream/

The Vegetarian Keto Diet

If you're reading this chapter, I can only assume it's because you weren't successful on the vegan keto diet. And you know what? That's perfectly acceptable. It is far more important by a mile that you are still trying to make an ethical keto diet work than just giving up altogether. This is where real strength comes from. Strength doesn't mean you're so incredible you succeed at every challenge on your first try. Strength means you keep trying until you succeed.

Make no mistake, the vegetarian keto diet is miles and miles easier than a vegan keto diet. Everything I've said in the entire book still applies to you. If you're vegetarian that means you're still forsaking all meat. All the rules of keto still apply including the 5% rule on carbs and the 20% rule on protein. All the benefits of a keto diet will still be yours, and all the possible side effects are still in place. But unlike the vegan keto diet, you get access to cheese, eggs, butter, and cream which make achieving ketosis so much easier.

Unlike the vegan diet where you have to rely on coconuts, avocados, and olives to get your much needed fat content, cheese and cream make this task so much easier. Avocado has 21 grams of fat in a 1 cup serving (146 grams). Cheddar cheese has 9 grams of fat in a 1 ounce serving (28 grams). With a little math we can see that cheddar cheese has double the fat content of avocado. Remember the keto diet isn't based on total calories but on calorie ratios. The more fat you eat, the more leeway you have with carbs.

Cream is also an excellent addition to a keto diet. While it may seem tempting to use in deserts, heavy cream is also an excellent addition to sauces and soups. Just 1 ounce of heavy cream, 1/8th of a cup, has 11 grams of fat and just .8 grams of carbs. When cooking with heavy cream, temper the cream before adding it to soups and sauces. Simply add a little bit of the soup or sauce to the cream to warm it up before you add it to the rest of the base or you'll cause curds to form.

Butter is an excellent food option when discussing keto. Butter has a whopping 12 grams of fat per serving with no carbs. It's extremely easy to prepare many keto vegetables in butter, or to create butter based sauces for vegetable noodles or mushrooms. Seriously, do not hesitate to load up on the butter. The more fat you can eat, the more likely you are to enter ketosis and stay in it.

Eggs are also an excellent addition to a keto diet, but not the staple that cheese and cream are. 1 large egg has 5 grams of fat and 6 grams of protein with just .6 grams of carbs. While that may seem like an ideal ratio of fat to carbs, you must remember excess protein in the keto diet is just as problematic as excess carbs. When you consume more protein than your body needs, it turns that excess protein into glucose which inhibits ketosis. The more active you are, the less likely you'll hit your protein limit, but it's still important to keep it in check. The best way to ensure that eating eggs enables ketosis is to eat them with cheese.

You may be wondering why I haven't included milk in the vegetarian keto section. It's high in protein, fat, and calcium which are three critical nutrients needed on the vegetarian keto diet. Milk is also loaded with a ton of sugar! Just 1 cup of milk has a whopping 12 grams of carbs in it. Even if you drank the very fatty whole milk, you would only get 8 grams of fat per serving compared to the 12 grams of carbs. There's no way that ratio works out in your favor, so it's best just to avoid milk altogether.

The Keto Diet

So, it's come to this. You found out a vegetarian diet isn't all it's cracked up to be. Don't get me wrong, I think a vegetarian diet is completely doable with a plethora of food options. Though people who grew up on a western diet may beg to differ. There's nothing wrong with stepping away from a vegetarian diet. We all do things our own way. Just like you shouldn't judge someone for being a vegetarian, you shouldn't judge someone who doesn't participate in those food practices. We all have different tolerances. Some of us struggle financially or lack the willpower. Some of us place a high priority on eating the tastiest food or having the most food selection available. There could be health reasons why a person can't be vegan or vegetarian. Regardless, the most important thing is to respect other people's choices.

Lucky for you though, the standard keto diet opens up a massive amount of tasty food opportunities to you. In addition to cheese, cream, eggs, and butter, you get access to some of the tastiest meats known to man. While some uninformed people will say you can eat any meat you want on the keto diet, and that is technically true, you want to focus on the fattiest meats possible. You must remember when eating meat that any excess protein you consume will be turned into glucose, and that will inhibit ketosis in your body. Below I have a list of the fattiest meats you should indulge in whenever possible.

Pork belly is far and away the best possible meat you can eat on keto. With a whopping 60 grams of fat, 10 grams of protein, and 0 grams of carbs, it is the ideal meat for keto and should be eaten whenever possible. Pork belly is an extremely savory cut of meat halfway between bacon and pork loin. The fat content make it extremely difficult to ruin the meat, even for inexperienced cooks. Fat is essential for keeping meat moist during the cooking process which keeps it tender and lends itself to a savory flavor. No meat even comes close to pork belly for keto.

Tied for second place is lamb chops and chicken thighs. Lamb chops have 29 grams of fat per serving, 17 grams of protein, and like all meat, 0 grams of carbs. Lamb chops are absolutely delicious, tasting similar to a very good steak but is really a taste unique to itself. Lamb chops should not be confused with mutton though. Mutton is very difficult to acquire in America, is very tough, and has a strong flavor. Stick with the lamb chops. Chicken thighs are probably a more realistic meal option for most people. Coming in at 25 grams of fat and 14 grams of protein per serving, chicken thighs are cheap, delicious, versatile, and available cut of eat. In a suburban area you should be able to find chicken thighs for less than a dollar a pound. They can be cooked in countless ways from grilling and deep frying, to baking and deboning then pan frying. Make sure you eat the skin to get all the available fat.

Coming in at third (or is it fourth?) is wonderful bacon. Ahhh bacon, what can't you do? Bacon has 3.3 grams of fat per slice and 3 grams of protein as well. Very few meats can boast of having a higher fat content than protein content. This is important for maintaining ketosis throughout your diet. You may be able to compensate with higher fat foods, but if you continually eat meat that's high in protein and low in fat, you run the risk of throwing off your calorie ratio. This is why I implore you to focus on these fatty meats. Bacon makes it so easy to stick to keto as it goes in just about anything. Sprinkle it on soups and salads. Add it to pasta. Eat it as a snack. Wrap it around chicken thighs when you bake them. It's easily the most versatile meat on the keto menu.

Finally, I want you to give some serious consideration to pork ribs. A serving of pork ribs contains 20 grams of fat and 21 grams of protein. Like bacon, there is a lot you can do with this fatty cut of meat. Forgo BBQ sauce and instead make your own spice rubs for your ribs. Feel free to cut them up and fry them for riblets. While the fat to protein ratio isn't as impressive as the previous meats, it's still one of the fattiest cuts of meat you can find.

Other than meat, there aren't many changes that come from leaving vegetarian keto for standard keto. I personally don't care how you get there, just as long as you get there. That's why I've given you information on all the possible diet combinations available in this book. If you succeed at vegan keto that's wonderful and truly a feat in itself. If you drop down to a standard keto diet, that's cool too. If you decide you just want to be vegan instead of doing keto, that's perfectly fine. Let's all just start respecting each others' diet choices.

If I've opened your eyes to new diet possibilities or taught you something you thought you already knew a lot about, then I have done my job. If I've given you a new mentality towards food, diets, or diet science, then I've done my job. If I've completely blown your mind with all this information, that's pretty cool too. Books teach us about the world. It's great you're consuming books for knowledge. That hunger for knowledge is a great thing. If books teach us about the world, then I think diets teach us about ourselves. On a diet, you learn what your body likes and doesn't like, you learn brand new things about food and what your tastes and sensibilities are. You're going to learn more about your body and health. You'll learn what it means to feel bad, but also what it means to feel good, to have more energy. You're going to learn how far your strength and willpower can take you. A diet is one of the ultimate tests a person can face. Unlike a race, or an academic test, they eventually end. You complete them and put them behind you. A diet is eternal. You're going to be eating and making food choices until the day you die. You're going to do this every single day, multiple times a day (you better be eating everyday, multiple times a day or I'm going to call your mom and tell her you haven't been eating). Diet is a test of willpower that is constantly in front of you everyday. Sometimes it's easy, other times it feels impossible. On a diet, you really learn what kind of strength of conviction you have, as that conviction will be tested everyday, multiple times a day. I wish you luck and strength in your journey. Happy dieting.

Vegan Keto Two Week Plan

Below I have put together a set of meals to accompany you through two weeks of the vegan ketogenic diet. This meal plan can easily be doubled over to create a months worth of meals. Feel free to mix and match options as you discover meal options you enjoy and dislike. Each set of meals will presented in a list of seven, you can do them in order or mix and match to your heart's content. Meal plans come from Dr. Jockers, Clean Keto Blog, Choose Veg, I Eat Keto, The Herbivore Post, Shape, Care2 and of course Pinterest.

Week 1

Breakfast

- Turmeric Coffee with Cocoa Butter
- Matcha Green Tea
- Dandelion Coffee with Coconut Milk (caffeine free)
- Tofu Scramble with Vegetables
- Chia Pudding
- Coconut Smoothie with Vanilla and Cinnamon
- Fried Spaghetti Squash Tots

Lunch

- Blueberry Protein Shake (vegetable protein, not whey)
- Chocolate Chia Smoothie (made with cacao)
- Avocado Based Salad
- Tofu and Cauliflower Stir Fry
- Seiten Negimaki (gluten seasoned like beef)
- Zucchini in Avocado Sauce
- Vegan Thai Soup with Mushroom and Ginger

Dinner

- Shiritaki Noodles with Tempeh and Veggies
- Garlic Basil Squash Spaghetti
- Creamy Coconut Guacamole Wraps
- Roasted Vegetable Masala
- Portabella Lettuce Wraps
- Cauliflower Pizza
- Walnut Chili

Week 2

Breakfast

- Vanilla Protein Powder Shake with Coconut Milk
- Vegan Pancakes
- Coconut Yogurt Bowl
- Chia and Hemp Seed Oatmeal
- Tofu French Toast Sticks
- Tofu Fritatta
- Avocado on Cauliflower Toast

Lunch

- Lupina Bean Falafel
- Green Curry Kale with Tempeh
- Grilled Portobello with Curried Spinach
- Grilled Veggies with Smoked Tofu in a Peanut Sauce
- Vegan Empanadas
- Tabbouleh (hemp heart salad)
- Zucchini Noodles with Vegan Cheese

Dinner

- Cauliflower Fried Rice
- Zucchini Lasagna
- Cucumber Mint Veggie Noodles
- Roasted Mushroom Medley
- Asian Brocoli Salad
- Roasted Brussels Sprouts with Vegan Cheese
- Egg Roll in a Bowl

Snacks

- Coconut Bacon Chips
- Almond Cheese
- Dehydrated Cauliflower
- Macadamia Nuts
- Crispy Salty Seaweed
- Ants on a Log with Humus and Sesame Seeds
- Keto Seed Crackers

Desserts

- Almond Butter Bars
- Coconut Milk Ice Cream
- Peanut Butter Truffles
- Raw Coconut Donuts
- Coconut Macaroons
- Dessert Almond Cheese
- Paleo Chocolate Hazelnut Cookies
- Peppermint Hemp Fat Fudge
- Raspberry Coconut Crack Bars
- Coconut Snowballs
- Carrot Cake Bites
- Protein Brownies